CKD STAGE 3 COOKBOOK FOR SENIORS

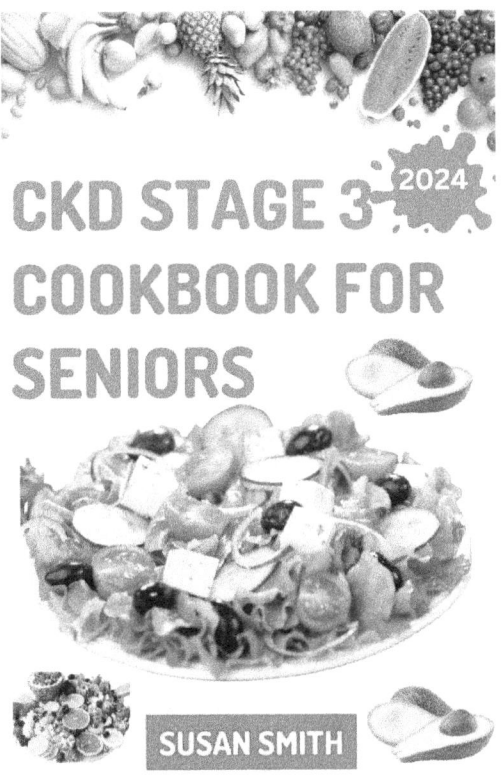

SUSAN SMITH

Copyright © 2024 by SUSAN SMITH

All rights reserved. No part of this publication may be reproduced, distributed, or transmitted in any form or by any means, including photocopying, recording, or other electronic or mechanical methods, without the prior written permission of the publisher, except in the case of brief quotations embodied in critical reviews and certain other non-commercial uses permitted by copyright law.

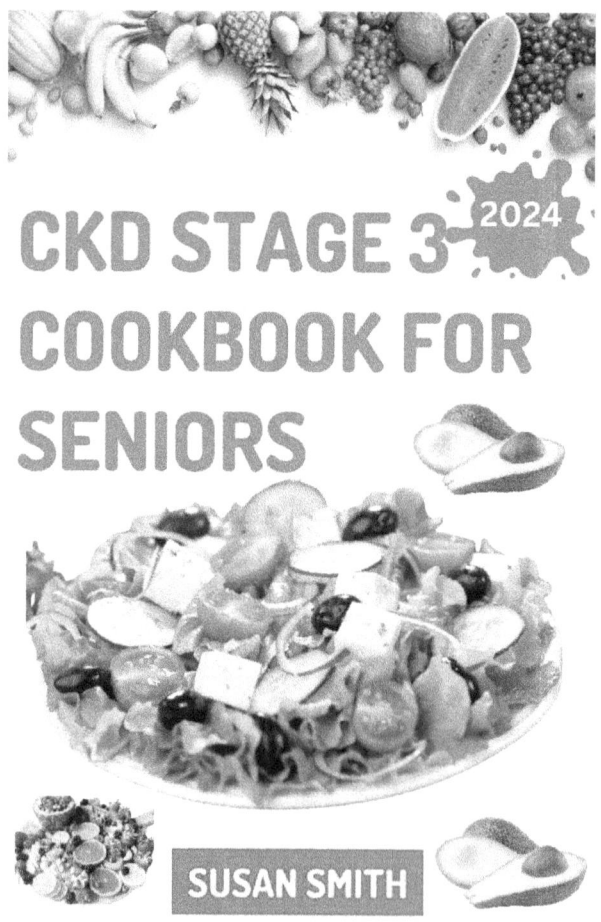

TABLE OF CONTENT

CHAPTER ONE: Introduction 7

   Understanding Chronic Kidney Disease (CKD) Stage 3 7

   1. Diagnosis and Definition: 7

   2. Causes and Risk Factors: 7

   3. Symptoms and Complications: 8

   4. Diagnostic Tests and Monitoring: 8

   5. Treatment and Management: 8

   6. Patient Education and Empowerment: 9

   Importance of Nutrition in Managing CKD 10

   Cooking and Eating Well with CKD 13

CHAPTER TWO: CKD Stage 3 Recipes 17

   CKD Stage 3 Breakfast Recipes 17

   1. Quinoa Breakfast Bowl: 17

   2. Vegetable Omelette: 18

   3. Greek Yogurt Parfait: 20

4. Sweet Potato Breakfast Hash: 21

5. Cottage Cheese and Fruit Bowl: 23

6. Veggie and Egg Muffin Cups: 24

7. Buckwheat Pancakes: 25

8. Spinach and Mushroom Frittata: 27

9. Millet Porridge with Berries: 29

10. Avocado Toast with Poached Egg: 30

CKD Stage 3 Lunch Recipes 32

1. Lemon Herb Baked Salmon: 32

2. Quinoa Salad with Chickpeas and Vegetables: 34

3. Turkey and Vegetable Stir-Fry: 35

4. Lentil and Vegetable Soup: 37

5. Tuna Salad Lettuce Wraps: 39

6. Eggplant and Chickpea Salad: 40

7. Turkey and Spinach Wrap: 42

8. Lentil and Vegetable Stir-Fry: 44

9. Mediterranean Chickpea Salad: 45

10. Grilled Chicken Caesar Salad: 47

CKD Stage 3 dinner Recipes 48

1. Baked Salmon with Roasted Vegetables: 48

2. Quinoa Stuffed Bell Peppers: 50

3. Baked Chicken and Vegetable Casserole: 52

4. Turkey and Quinoa Stuffed Acorn Squash: 54

5. Lemon Herb Baked Cod: 56

6. Vegetable and Lentil Curry: 58

7. Quinoa and Vegetable Stir-Fry: 60

8. Baked Eggplant Parmesan: 62

9. Lemon Garlic Shrimp with Asparagus: 64

10. Turkey and Vegetable Skillet: 65

CKD Stage 3 Snack Recipes 67

1. Baked Sweet Potato Chips: 67

2. Greek Yogurt with Berries and Almonds: 68

3. Cucumber and Hummus Bites: 69

4. Apple and Almond Butter Slices: 70

5. Rice Cake with Avocado and Tomato: 72

6. Cottage Cheese and Pineapple Spears: 73

7. Tuna Cucumber Bites: 74

8. Rice Paper Spring Rolls: 75

9. Egg Salad Lettuce Wraps: 77

10. Caprese Skewers: 78

CONCLUSION 80

Common Concerns About Diet and CKD Stage 3 80

Lifestyle Adjustments for Better Kidney Health 82

CHAPTER ONE: Introduction

Understanding Chronic Kidney Disease (CKD) Stage 3

Chronic Kidney Disease (CKD) Stage 3 marks a pivotal point in the progression of renal dysfunction, where kidney function has declined to a moderate level.

Understanding CKD Stage 3 is essential for individuals affected by this condition, as well as for their caregivers and healthcare providers. This stage signifies a critical juncture where proactive measures can significantly influence disease management and progression.

1. Diagnosis and Definition:

CKD Stage 3 is diagnosed based on an estimated Glomerular Filtration Rate (eGFR) ranging from 30 to 59 milliliters per minute per 1.73 meters squared. This stage is characterized by a moderate decline in kidney function, where the kidneys are still able to perform some of their essential functions, but their efficiency is notably reduced.

2. Causes and Risk Factors:

Various factors contribute to the development and progression of CKD Stage 3.

Common causes include hypertension, diabetes mellitus, glomerulonephritis, polycystic kidney disease, and autoimmune diseases such as lupus nephritis. Other risk factors include aging, obesity, smoking, family history of kidney disease, and certain medications.

3. Symptoms and Complications:

In CKD Stage 3, individuals may start to experience symptoms such as fatigue, fluid retention, swelling (edema), changes in urination frequency and color, hypertension, anemia, and bone disorders.

If left unmanaged, CKD Stage 3 can progress to more severe stages, leading to complications such as cardiovascular disease, kidney failure (end-stage renal disease), electrolyte imbalances, and metabolic acidosis.

4. Diagnostic Tests and Monitoring:

To diagnose and monitor CKD Stage 3, healthcare providers may conduct various tests, including blood tests to measure serum creatinine and estimate the eGFR, urine tests to assess proteinuria and hematuria, imaging studies such as ultrasound or CT scans, and kidney biopsy in some cases.

5. Treatment and Management:

The management of CKD Stage 3 aims to slow disease progression, alleviate symptoms, and reduce the risk of complications.

Lifestyle modifications, including dietary changes (such as reducing sodium, phosphorus, and potassium intake), regular exercise, smoking cessation, and weight management, play a crucial role.

Medications may be prescribed to control blood pressure, manage diabetes, treat anemia, and address other underlying conditions contributing to CKD progression. In some cases, referral to a nephrologist and consideration of renal replacement therapy options may be necessary.

6. Patient Education and Empowerment:

Educating individuals with CKD Stage 3 about their condition, treatment options, and lifestyle modifications is paramount. Empowering patients to actively participate in their care, adhere to medication regimens, monitor their symptoms, and make informed decisions regarding their health can improve outcomes and quality of life.

Understanding CKD Stage 3 involves recognizing its causes, symptoms, diagnostic criteria, and management strategies. With early detection, appropriate interventions, and ongoing monitoring, individuals with CKD Stage 3 can better manage their condition, delay disease progression, and maintain optimal kidney function for as long as possible.

Collaboration between patients, caregivers, and healthcare providers is essential in navigating the complexities of CKD Stage 3 and promoting kidney health and overall well-being.

Importance of Nutrition in Managing CKD

Nutrition plays a critical role in managing Chronic Kidney Disease (CKD) by helping to control symptoms, slow the progression of the disease, and improve overall health and well-being. Here's a comprehensive overview of the importance of nutrition in managing CKD:

1. Control of Protein Intake:

In CKD, the kidneys may struggle to filter waste products from the blood, leading to a buildup of urea and other nitrogenous waste products. Reducing protein intake can help lessen the burden on the kidneys and decrease the accumulation of waste products in the body.

However, it's essential to ensure that individuals with CKD still consume enough high-quality protein to maintain muscle mass and support overall health.

2. Monitoring Sodium (Salt) Intake:

Excess sodium can lead to fluid retention and hypertension, which are common complications of CKD. Managing sodium intake is crucial for controlling blood pressure and reducing the risk of fluid overload and swelling (edema).

Limiting processed and packaged foods, which are often high in sodium, and cooking with herbs and spices instead of salt can help individuals with CKD maintain a low-sodium diet.

3. Regulation of Potassium and Phosphorus Levels:

Advanced stages of CKD, the kidneys may struggle to regulate potassium and phosphorus levels in the blood, leading to hyperkalemia and hyperphosphatemia.

Monitoring and managing the intake of potassium- and phosphorus-rich foods, such as bananas, oranges, tomatoes, dairy products, and processed meats, can help prevent complications such as abnormal heart rhythms and bone disorders.

4. Fluid Management:

Individuals with CKD may experience fluid retention, which can lead to swelling, high blood pressure, and shortness of breath. Monitoring fluid intake and limiting fluids, especially in later stages of CKD, can help prevent fluid overload and alleviate symptoms. Healthcare providers may recommend specific fluid restrictions based on individual needs and stage of CKD.

5. Attention to Micronutrient Needs:

CKD can affect the body's ability to absorb and utilize certain vitamins and minerals, such as vitamin D, calcium, iron, and B vitamins. Monitoring and supplementing as necessary can help prevent deficiencies and support overall health. Additionally, some individuals with CKD may require erythropoiesis-stimulating agents (ESAs) or iron supplements to manage anemia.

6. Individualized Nutrition Counseling:

Nutrition needs can vary widely among individuals with CKD based on factors such as stage of the disease, age, gender, weight, activity level, and presence of other medical conditions.

Individualized nutrition counseling from a registered dietitian or healthcare provider specializing in renal nutrition is essential for developing personalized meal plans, addressing dietary restrictions and preferences, and optimizing nutritional intake.

7. Supportive Role in Overall Health and Well-being:

Nutrition plays a pivotal role in supporting overall health and well-being in individuals with CKD. A well-balanced diet that focuses on whole, nutrient-rich foods can help boost energy levels, improve immune function, promote healing, and enhance quality of life for individuals living with CKD.

Nutrition is a cornerstone of CKD management, with dietary interventions playing a crucial role in controlling symptoms, slowing disease progression, and improving outcomes. By following a renal-friendly diet tailored to their individual needs, individuals with CKD can better manage their condition, optimize kidney function, and maintain overall health and well-being.

Cooking and Eating Well with CKD

Cooking and eating well with Chronic Kidney Disease (CKD) require careful consideration of dietary restrictions and nutritional needs to support kidney health and overall well-being. Here are comprehensive tips for cooking and eating well with CKD:

1. Understand Dietary Restrictions:

Familiarize yourself with the dietary restrictions specific to CKD, including limitations on protein, sodium, potassium, and phosphorus intake.

Consult with a registered dietitian specializing in renal nutrition to develop a personalized meal plan tailored to your individual needs and stage of CKD.

2. Choose Kidney-Friendly Foods:

Opt for fresh, whole foods whenever possible, including fruits, vegetables, whole grains, lean proteins, and healthy fats.

Select low-phosphorus and low-potassium options such as apples, berries, cabbage, cauliflower, green beans, rice, and pasta.

Use herbs, spices, and lemon juice to flavor dishes instead of salt to reduce sodium intake.

3. Practice Portion Control:

Be mindful of portion sizes to avoid overconsumption of nutrients that need to be limited, such as protein, sodium, and phosphorus.

Use measuring cups, spoons, and kitchen scales to portion out foods accurately, especially high-protein items like meat, poultry, and fish.

4. Cook with Kidney-Friendly Methods:

Choose cooking methods that minimize the need for added fats and oils, such as baking, grilling, broiling, steaming, and sautéing with minimal oil.

Avoid frying foods, as it can increase their fat content and contribute to excess calorie consumption.

5. Monitor Fluid Intake:

Keep track of your fluid intake throughout the day to adhere to any fluid restrictions recommended by your healthcare provider.

Sip fluids slowly and avoid drinking large amounts of fluid all at once to prevent fluid overload and swelling (edema).

6. Read Food Labels:

Pay close attention to food labels when grocery shopping to identify hidden sources of sodium, potassium, and phosphorus in packaged and processed foods.

Look for products labeled "low-sodium," "low-potassium," or "phosphate-free" when available.

7. Plan Meals in Advance:

Plan your meals and snacks in advance to ensure they align with your dietary restrictions and nutritional goals.

Batch cook and prepare meals ahead of time to save time and reduce the temptation of choosing convenience foods that may not be kidney-friendly.

8. Experiment with Kidney-Friendly Recipes:

Explore a variety of kidney-friendly recipes that incorporate fresh, whole ingredients and flavorful herbs and spices.

Get creative in the kitchen by trying new cooking techniques and flavor combinations to keep meals interesting and satisfying.

9. Stay Connected with Support Networks:

Join online communities or support groups for individuals living with CKD to share experiences, recipes, and tips for managing the condition.

Stay connected with your healthcare team, including your nephrologist and dietitian, to receive ongoing guidance and support in managing your diet and overall health.

10. Practice Mindful Eating:

Eat slowly, chew food thoroughly, and savor each bite to promote digestion and enhance satisfaction.

Pay attention to hunger and fullness cues to avoid overeating and maintain a healthy weight.

By following these comprehensive tips for cooking and eating well with CKD, you can support kidney health, manage symptoms, and improve overall well-being while enjoying delicious and nourishing meals.

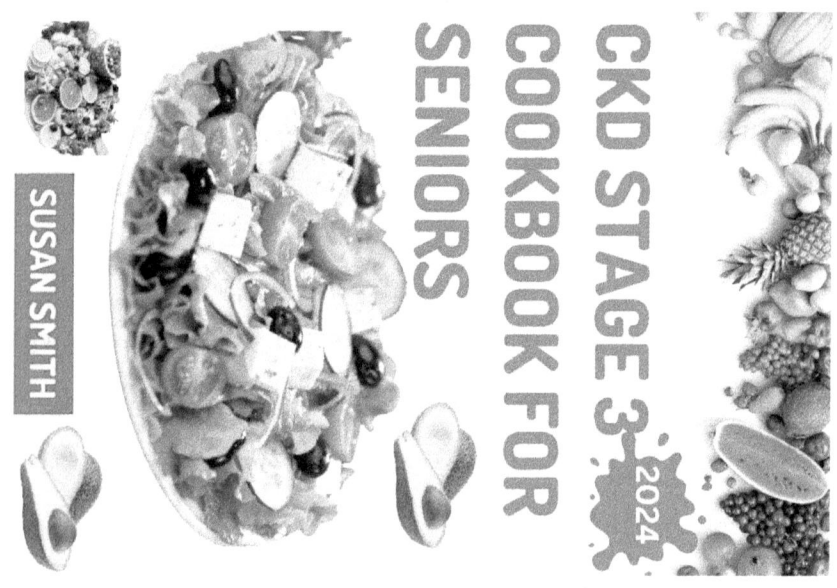

CHAPTER TWO: CKD Stage 3 Recipes

CKD Stage 3 Breakfast Recipes

1. Quinoa Breakfast Bowl:

Ingredients:

- 1/2 cup cooked quinoa

- 1/4 cup sliced strawberries

- 1/4 cup blueberries

- 1 tablespoon chopped almonds

- 1 tablespoon ground flaxseeds

- 1/4 teaspoon cinnamon

- 1/4 cup unsweetened almond milk (or any milk of choice)

Instructions:

- Cook quinoa according to package instructions and let it cool slightly.

- In a bowl, combine cooked quinoa, sliced strawberries, blueberries, chopped almonds, ground flaxseeds, and cinnamon.

- Pour almond milk over the top and stir to combine.

- Serve immediately and enjoy!

Health Benefits:

Quinoa is a high-protein grain alternative that provides essential amino acids without contributing to high levels of phosphorus and potassium.

• Berries are rich in antioxidants, fiber, and vitamin C, which support overall health and may help reduce inflammation.

• Almonds and flaxseeds are excellent sources of healthy fats, fiber, and protein, promoting satiety and heart health.

Preparation Time: Approximately 15 minutes.

2. Vegetable Omelette

Ingredients:

• 2 large eggs

• 1/4 cup diced bell peppers

• 1/4 cup diced onions

• 1/4 cup diced mushrooms

• 1/4 cup chopped spinach

• 1 tablespoon olive oil

• Salt and pepper to taste

Instructions:

- In a bowl, beat the eggs and season with salt and pepper.
- Heat olive oil in a non-stick skillet over medium heat.
- Add diced bell peppers, onions, and mushrooms to the skillet and sauté until softened.
- Add chopped spinach to the skillet and cook until wilted.
- Pour the beaten eggs over the vegetables and cook until the edges start to set.
- Using a spatula, gently lift the edges of the omelette and tilt the skillet to allow the uncooked eggs to flow underneath.
- Once the omelette is cooked through, fold it in half and transfer to a plate.
- Serve hot and enjoy!

Health Benefits:

- Eggs are an excellent source of high-quality protein and essential nutrients like vitamin D and B vitamins.
- Vegetables like bell peppers, onions, mushrooms, and spinach provide vitamins, minerals, and antioxidants while being low in phosphorus and potassium.

Preparation Time: Approximately 20 minutes.

3. Greek Yogurt Parfait:

Ingredients:

- 1/2 cup low-fat Greek yogurt
- 1/4 cup sliced strawberries
- 1/4 cup diced mango
- 1 tablespoon chopped walnuts
- 1 tablespoon honey (optional)
- 1/4 teaspoon vanilla extract

Instructions:

- In a bowl, mix together Greek yogurt, vanilla extract, and honey (if using).
- In a serving glass or bowl, layer the Greek yogurt mixture with sliced strawberries, diced mango, and chopped walnuts.
- Repeat the layers until all ingredients are used, ending with a layer of fruit and nuts on top.

Serve immediately or refrigerate until ready to eat.

Health Benefits:

• Greek yogurt is high in protein and calcium, providing essential nutrients without contributing to high levels of phosphorus and potassium.

• Strawberries and mangoes are rich in vitamins, minerals, and antioxidants, supporting overall health and immune function.

• Walnuts are a good source of heart-healthy fats and omega-3 fatty acids, promoting cardiovascular health.

Preparation Time: Approximately 10 minutes.

4. Sweet Potato Breakfast Hash:

Ingredients:

• 1 small sweet potato, peeled and diced

• 1/4 cup diced bell peppers

• 1/4 cup diced onions

• 1/4 cup cooked black beans (rinsed and drained)

• 1 tablespoon olive oil

• Salt and pepper to taste

• 1 tablespoon chopped parsley (optional)

Instructions:

- Heat olive oil in a skillet over medium heat.

- Add diced sweet potato to the skillet and cook until tender and lightly browned, about 8-10 minutes.

- Add diced bell peppers and onions to the skillet and cook until softened.

- Stir in cooked black beans and continue cooking until heated through.

- Season with salt and pepper to taste and garnish with chopped parsley if desired.

- Serve hot and enjoy!

Health Benefits:

- Sweet potatoes are rich in vitamins A and C, fiber, and antioxidants, supporting immune function and heart health.

- Black beans are an excellent source of plant-based protein and fiber, promoting satiety and digestive health.

- Bell peppers and onions add flavor, color, and additional vitamins and minerals to the dish.

Preparation Time: Approximately 20 minutes.

5. Cottage Cheese and Fruit Bowl:

Ingredients:

- 1/2 cup low-fat cottage cheese
- 1/4 cup diced pineapple
- 1/4 cup diced kiwi
- 1 tablespoon unsalted sunflower seeds
- 1 tablespoon honey (optional)
- 1/4 teaspoon cinnamon

Instructions:

- In a bowl, scoop the cottage cheese.
- Top the cottage cheese with diced pineapple and kiwi.
- Sprinkle unsalted sunflower seeds over the fruit.
- Drizzle honey over the top if desired.
- Sprinkle with cinnamon for added flavor.
- Serve immediately and enjoy!

Health Benefits:

- Cottage cheese is a good source of protein and calcium, essential for muscle and bone health.

Pineapple and kiwi are low-potassium fruits rich in vitamins C and K, which support immune function and bone health.

Sunflower seeds provide healthy fats and protein, adding crunch and flavor to the dish.

Preparation Time: Approximately 5 minutes.

6. Veggie and Egg Muffin Cups:

Ingredients:

- 4 large eggs

- 1/4 cup diced tomatoes

- 1/4 cup diced zucchini

- 1/4 cup diced bell peppers

- 2 tablespoons grated Parmesan cheese

- Salt and pepper to taste

Instructions:

- Preheat the oven to 350°F (175°C) and lightly grease a muffin tin.

- In a bowl, beat the eggs and season with salt and pepper.

- Stir in diced tomatoes, zucchini, bell peppers, and grated Parmesan cheese.

- Pour the egg mixture evenly into the muffin tin, filling each cup about two-thirds full.

- Bake in the preheated oven for 20-25 minutes, or until the egg muffins are set and lightly golden on top.

- Allow the muffins to cool slightly before removing them from the tin.

- Serve warm or at room temperature.

Health Benefits:

- Eggs are a complete protein source and provide essential nutrients like vitamin D and B vitamins.

- Tomatoes, zucchini, and bell peppers add vitamins, minerals, and antioxidants to the dish while being low in potassium.

- Parmesan cheese adds flavor and a calcium boost to support bone health.

Preparation Time: Approximately 30 minutes.

7. Buckwheat Pancakes:

Ingredients:

- 1/2 cup buckwheat flour

- 1/4 teaspoon baking powder

- 1/4 teaspoon cinnamon
- 1/2 cup unsweetened almond milk (or any milk of choice)
- 1 tablespoon unsweetened applesauce
- 1 teaspoon vanilla extract
- Fresh berries for topping (optional)
- Maple syrup or honey for drizzling (optional)

Instructions:

- In a mixing bowl, whisk together buckwheat flour, baking powder, and cinnamon.
- Stir in almond milk, unsweetened applesauce, and vanilla extract until well combined.
- Heat a non-stick skillet over medium heat and lightly grease with cooking spray or oil.
- Pour 1/4 cup of batter onto the skillet for each pancake.
- Cook until bubbles form on the surface, then flip and cook until golden brown on both sides.
- Serve warm with fresh berries and a drizzle of maple syrup or honey if desired.

Health Benefits:

• Buckwheat flour is a gluten-free whole grain rich in fiber, protein, and minerals like magnesium and iron.

• Unsweetened applesauce adds moisture and natural sweetness to the pancakes without added sugars.

• Berries are low-potassium fruits packed with antioxidants and vitamins, supporting overall health.

Preparation Time: Approximately 15 minutes.

8. Spinach and Mushroom Frittata:

Ingredients:

• 4 large eggs

• 1 cup chopped spinach

• 1/2 cup sliced mushrooms

• 1/4 cup diced onions

• 2 tablespoons grated Parmesan cheese

• Salt and pepper to taste

• 1 tablespoon olive oil

Instructions:

- Preheat the oven to 350°F (175°C).

- In a bowl, beat the eggs and season with salt and pepper.

- Heat olive oil in an oven-safe skillet over medium heat.

- Add diced onions and sliced mushrooms to the skillet and cook until softened.

- Add chopped spinach to the skillet and cook until wilted.

- Pour the beaten eggs over the vegetables in the skillet.

- Sprinkle grated Parmesan cheese over the top.

- Transfer the skillet to the preheated oven and bake for 15-20 minutes, or until the frittata is set and golden brown on top.

- Slice into wedges and serve hot.

Health Benefits:

- Spinach is a nutrient-dense leafy green rich in vitamins A, C, and K, as well as iron and folate.

- Mushrooms add savory flavor and provide vitamins, minerals, and antioxidants.

- Eggs are a complete protein source and supply essential nutrients like vitamin D and B vitamins.

Preparation Time: Approximately 30 minutes.

9. Millet Porridge with Berries:

Ingredients:

• 1/2 cup millet

• 1 1/2 cups water

• 1/2 cup low-fat milk or unsweetened almond milk

• 1/4 teaspoon cinnamon

• 1/4 cup mixed berries (such as blueberries, raspberries, or strawberries)

• 1 tablespoon chopped walnuts (optional)

• 1 tablespoon honey or maple syrup (optional)

Instructions:

• Rinse the millet under cold water.

• In a saucepan, bring the water to a boil, then add the rinsed millet.

• Reduce the heat to low, cover, and simmer for 15-20 minutes, or until the millet is tender and the water is absorbed.

• Stir in the milk and cinnamon and continue to cook for another 5-10 minutes, until the mixture thickens to a porridge-like consistency.

- Remove from heat and let it cool slightly.

- Serve the millet porridge topped with mixed berries and chopped walnuts.

- Drizzle with honey or maple syrup if desired.

Health Benefits:

- Millet is a gluten-free whole grain rich in fiber and minerals like magnesium and phosphorus.

- Berries are low-potassium fruits packed with antioxidants and vitamins, supporting overall health and immune function.

- Walnuts add a crunch and provide heart-healthy fats like omega-3 fatty acids.

Preparation Time: Approximately 30 minutes.

10. Avocado Toast with Poached Egg:

Ingredients:

- 1 slice whole grain bread

- 1/2 ripe avocado, mashed

- 1 large egg

- Salt and pepper to taste

- Red pepper flakes for garnish (optional)

- Fresh parsley for garnish (optional)

Instructions:

- Toast the whole grain bread until golden brown.

- Spread the mashed avocado evenly on the toast.

- In a saucepan, bring water to a simmer, then reduce the heat to low.

- Crack the egg into a small bowl, then gently slide it into the simmering water.

- Poach the egg for 3-4 minutes, until the whites are set but the yolk is still runny.

- Using a slotted spoon, carefully remove the poached egg from the water and place it on top of the avocado toast.

- Season with salt, pepper, red pepper flakes, and fresh parsley if desired.

- Serve immediately and enjoy!

Health Benefits:

- Whole grain bread provides fiber and complex carbohydrates for sustained energy.

- Avocado is rich in heart-healthy fats, fiber, and potassium.

- Eggs are a complete protein source and supply essential nutrients like vitamin D and B vitamins.

Preparation Time: Approximately 15 minutes.

CKD Stage 3 Lunch Recipes

1. Lemon Herb Baked Salmon:

Ingredients:

- 1 salmon fillet (4-6 ounces)

- 1 tablespoon olive oil

- 1 tablespoon freshly squeezed lemon juice

- 1 clove garlic, minced

- 1 teaspoon fresh thyme leaves (or 1/2 teaspoon dried thyme)

- Salt and pepper to taste

- Lemon slices for garnish (optional)

- Fresh parsley for garnish (optional)

Instructions:

- Preheat the oven to 375°F (190°C) and line a baking dish with parchment paper.

- Place the salmon fillet in the baking dish.

- In a small bowl, whisk together olive oil, lemon juice, minced garlic, and thyme.

- Pour the lemon herb mixture over the salmon fillet, coating it evenly.

- Season the salmon with salt and pepper to taste.

- Bake in the preheated oven for 12-15 minutes, or until the salmon is cooked through and flakes easily with a fork.

- Remove from the oven and let it rest for a few minutes.

- Garnish with lemon slices and fresh parsley if desired.

- Serve hot and enjoy!

Health Benefits:

- Salmon is a rich source of omega-3 fatty acids, which are beneficial for heart health and may help reduce inflammation.

- Olive oil provides healthy fats and antioxidants, promoting cardiovascular health.

- Lemon juice adds a burst of flavor and provides vitamin C, supporting immune function.

Preparation Time: Approximately 20 minutes.

2. Quinoa Salad with Chickpeas and Vegetables:

Ingredients:

- 1/2 cup quinoa

- 1 cup water or low-sodium vegetable broth

- 1/2 cup cooked chickpeas (rinsed and drained if canned)

- 1/4 cup diced cucumbers

- 1/4 cup diced bell peppers

- 1/4 cup halved cherry tomatoes

- 2 tablespoons chopped fresh parsley

- 1 tablespoon extra-virgin olive oil

- 1 tablespoon freshly squeezed lemon juice

- Salt and pepper to taste

Instructions:

- Rinse the quinoa under cold water.

- In a saucepan, bring water or vegetable broth to a boil.

- Add the rinsed quinoa to the saucepan, reduce the heat to low, cover, and simmer for 15-20 minutes, or until the quinoa is tender and the liquid is absorbed.

- Fluff the cooked quinoa with a fork and let it cool slightly.

- In a large bowl, combine cooked quinoa, chickpeas, diced cucumbers, bell peppers, cherry tomatoes, and chopped parsley.

- In a small bowl, whisk together olive oil and lemon juice to make the dressing.

- Pour the dressing over the quinoa salad and toss to coat evenly.

- Season with salt and pepper to taste.

- Serve immediately or refrigerate until ready to eat.

Health Benefits:

- Quinoa is a gluten-free whole grain rich in protein, fiber, and essential nutrients.

- Chickpeas provide plant-based protein and fiber, promoting satiety and digestive health.

- Vegetables like cucumbers, bell peppers, and tomatoes are low in potassium and rich in vitamins, minerals, and antioxidants.

Preparation Time: Approximately 30 minutes.

3. Turkey and Vegetable Stir-Fry:

Ingredients:

- 4 ounces lean turkey breast, thinly sliced

- 1 cup mixed vegetables (such as bell peppers, broccoli, carrots, and snap peas)
- 1 tablespoon low-sodium soy sauce
- 1 tablespoon olive oil
- 1 clove garlic, minced
- 1 teaspoon grated ginger
- 2 tablespoons chopped green onions (optional)
- Sesame seeds for garnish (optional)
- Cooked brown rice for serving

Instructions:

- Heat olive oil in a large skillet or wok over medium-high heat.
- Add minced garlic and grated ginger to the skillet and sauté for 1 minute.
- Add thinly sliced turkey breast to the skillet and cook until browned and cooked through.
- Add mixed vegetables to the skillet and stir-fry until tender-crisp.
- Stir in low-sodium soy sauce and chopped green onions (if using), and cook for an additional 1-2 minutes.
- Remove from heat and garnish with sesame seeds if desired.

- Serve hot over cooked brown rice.

Health Benefits:

- Lean turkey breast is a good source of high-quality protein, essential for muscle maintenance and repair.

- Mixed vegetables provide vitamins, minerals, and antioxidants while being low in potassium.

- Brown rice is a whole grain rich in fiber, promoting digestive health and providing sustained energy.

Preparation Time: Approximately 20 minutes.

4. Lentil and Vegetable Soup:

Ingredients:

- 1/2 cup dried green or brown lentils, rinsed and drained

- 4 cups low-sodium vegetable broth

- 1 cup diced carrots

- 1 cup diced celery

- 1 cup diced onions

- 2 cloves garlic, minced

- 1 teaspoon dried thyme

- 1 bay leaf

- Salt and pepper to taste

- Fresh parsley for garnish (optional)

Instructions:

- In a large pot, combine dried lentils, low-sodium vegetable broth, diced carrots, celery, onions, minced garlic, dried thyme, and bay leaf.

- Bring the soup to a boil, then reduce the heat to low and simmer, covered, for 20-25 minutes, or until the lentils and vegetables are tender.

- Season the soup with salt and pepper to taste.

- Remove the bay leaf before serving.

- Ladle the soup into bowls and garnish with fresh parsley if desired.

- Serve hot and enjoy!

Health Benefits:

- Lentils are a plant-based source of protein and fiber, promoting satiety and digestive health.

- Vegetables like carrots, celery, and onions add vitamins, minerals, and antioxidants to the soup while being low in potassium.

- Vegetable broth provides flavor and hydration without added sodium.

Preparation Time: Approximately 30 minutes.

5. Tuna Salad Lettuce Wraps:

Ingredients:

- 1 can (5 ounces) tuna, drained
- 1/4 cup diced cucumber
- 1/4 cup diced red bell pepper
- 2 tablespoons diced red onion
- 2 tablespoons chopped fresh parsley
- 2 tablespoons plain Greek yogurt
- 1 tablespoon lemon juice
- Salt and pepper to taste
- 4 large lettuce leaves (such as romaine or butter lettuce)

Instructions:

- In a bowl, mix together drained tuna, diced cucumber, diced red bell pepper, diced red onion, chopped fresh parsley, plain Greek yogurt, and lemon juice.

- Season with salt and pepper to taste and mix until well combined.

- Place a spoonful of the tuna salad mixture onto each lettuce leaf.

- Roll up the lettuce leaves to form wraps.

- Serve immediately or refrigerate until ready to eat.

Health Benefits:

- Tuna is a lean source of protein and omega-3 fatty acids, supporting heart health and providing essential nutrients.

- Vegetables like cucumber, red bell pepper, and red onion add vitamins, minerals, and antioxidants to the salad while being low in potassium.

- Greek yogurt provides creaminess and protein without adding excessive phosphorus or potassium.

Preparation Time: Approximately 10 minutes.

6. Eggplant and Chickpea Salad:

Ingredients:

- 1 small eggplant, diced

- 1 can (15 ounces) chickpeas, rinsed and drained

- 1/4 cup diced tomatoes

- 1/4 cup diced red onion

- 2 tablespoons chopped fresh mint
- 2 tablespoons extra-virgin olive oil
- 1 tablespoon balsamic vinegar
- Salt and pepper to taste

Instructions:

- Preheat the oven to 400°F (200°C) and line a baking sheet with parchment paper.
- Place diced eggplant on the prepared baking sheet and drizzle with olive oil.
- Roast in the preheated oven for 20-25 minutes, or until the eggplant is tender and lightly browned.
- In a large bowl, combine roasted eggplant, chickpeas, diced tomatoes, diced red onion, and chopped fresh mint.
- Drizzle with balsamic vinegar and toss to coat evenly.
- Season with salt and pepper to taste.
- Serve the salad at room temperature or chilled.

Health Benefits:

• Eggplant is low in potassium and provides fiber and antioxidants, supporting digestive health and heart health.

• Chickpeas are a good source of plant-based protein and fiber, promoting satiety and stabilizing blood sugar levels.

• Tomatoes add vitamins, minerals, and antioxidants to the salad while being low in potassium.

Preparation Time: Approximately 30 minutes.

7. Turkey and Spinach Wraps

Ingredients:

• 4 ounces cooked turkey breast, sliced

• 1 whole wheat or low-sodium wrap

• 1/4 cup baby spinach leaves

• 1/4 cup shredded carrots

• 1/4 cup diced tomatoes

• 1 tablespoon hummus

• 1 teaspoon Dijon mustard

• Salt and pepper to taste

Instructions:

- Lay the whole wheat wrap on a clean surface.
- Spread hummus evenly over the wrap, leaving a small border around the edges.
- Drizzle Dijon mustard over the hummus.
- Layer sliced turkey breast, baby spinach leaves, shredded carrots, and diced tomatoes on top of the hummus.
- Season with salt and pepper to taste.
- Roll up the wrap tightly, tucking in the sides as you go.
- Slice the wrap in half diagonally and serve.

Health Benefits:

- Turkey breast is a lean source of protein and provides essential amino acids for muscle maintenance and repair.
- Spinach is low in potassium and rich in vitamins A and K, promoting eye health and bone health.
- Whole wheat wraps provide complex carbohydrates and fiber, helping to stabilize blood sugar levels and promote digestive health.

Preparation Time: Approximately 10 minutes.

8. Lentil and Vegetable Stir-Fry:

Ingredients:

- 1/2 cup dried lentils, rinsed and drained
- 1 cup low-sodium vegetable broth
- 1 cup mixed vegetables (such as bell peppers, broccoli, carrots, and snap peas)
- 2 tablespoons low-sodium soy sauce
- 1 tablespoon olive oil
- 1 clove garlic, minced
- 1 teaspoon grated ginger
- 1 tablespoon chopped green onions (optional)
- Cooked brown rice for serving

Instructions:

- In a saucepan, combine dried lentils and low-sodium vegetable broth. Bring to a boil, then reduce heat, cover, and simmer for 20-25 minutes, or until lentils are tender.
- In a large skillet or wok, heat olive oil over medium-high heat. Add minced garlic and grated ginger, and cook for 1 minute.
- Add mixed vegetables to the skillet and stir-fry until tender-crisp.

- Add cooked lentils and low-sodium soy sauce to the skillet, and toss to combine.

- Cook for an additional 2-3 minutes, until heated through.

- Garnish with chopped green onions if desired.

- Serve the lentil and vegetable stir-fry over cooked brown rice.

Health Benefits:

- Lentils are a good source of plant-based protein and provide fiber, promoting satiety and digestive health.

- Mixed vegetables offer a variety of vitamins, minerals, and antioxidants while being low in potassium.

- Brown rice provides complex carbohydrates and fiber, helping to stabilize blood sugar levels and promote digestive health.

Preparation Time: Approximately 30 minutes.

9. Mediterranean Chickpea Salad:

Ingredients:

- 1 can (15 ounces) chickpeas, rinsed and drained

- 1 cup diced cucumbers

- 1 cup halved cherry tomatoes

- 1/4 cup diced red onion

- 1/4 cup chopped fresh parsley

- 2 tablespoons extra-virgin olive oil

- 1 tablespoon red wine vinegar

- 1 teaspoon dried oregano

- Salt and pepper to taste

- Crumbled feta cheese for garnish (optional)

Instructions:

- In a large bowl, combine chickpeas, diced cucumbers, halved cherry tomatoes, diced red onion, and chopped fresh parsley.

- In a small bowl, whisk together extra-virgin olive oil, red wine vinegar, dried oregano, salt, and pepper to make the dressing.

- Pour the dressing over the chickpea salad and toss to coat evenly.

- Garnish with crumbled feta cheese if desired.

- Serve chilled or at room temperature.

Health Benefits:

- Chickpeas are a good source of plant-based protein and fiber, promoting satiety and digestive health.

- Vegetables like cucumbers, tomatoes, and onions provide vitamins, minerals, and antioxidants while being low in potassium.

- Extra-virgin olive oil is rich in heart-healthy monounsaturated fats and antioxidants, supporting cardiovascular health.

Preparation Time: Approximately 15 minutes.

10. Grilled Chicken Caesar Salad:

Ingredients:

- 4 ounces grilled chicken breast, sliced

- 2 cups chopped romaine lettuce

- 1/4 cup diced tomatoes

- 2 tablespoons shredded Parmesan cheese

- 2 tablespoons Caesar dressing (low-sodium or homemade)

- 1 tablespoon croutons (optional)

- Lemon wedges for garnish (optional)

Instructions:

- In a large bowl, combine chopped romaine lettuce, diced tomatoes, and shredded Parmesan cheese.

- Add sliced grilled chicken breast to the bowl.

- Drizzle Caesar dressing over the salad and toss to coat evenly.

- Garnish with croutons if desired.

• Serve immediately with lemon wedges on the side.

Health Benefits:

• Grilled chicken breast is a lean source of protein and provides essential amino acids for muscle maintenance and repair.

• Romaine lettuce is low in potassium and rich in vitamins A and K, promoting eye health and bone health.

• Parmesan cheese adds flavor and provides calcium and protein while being low in phosphorus.

Preparation Time: Approximately 20 minutes.

CKD Stage 3 dinner Recipes

1. Baked Salmon with Roasted Vegetables:

Ingredients:

• 1 salmon fillet (4-6 ounces)

• 1 cup mixed vegetables (such as bell peppers, zucchini, and carrots), chopped

• 1 tablespoon olive oil

• 1/2 teaspoon dried Italian seasoning

• Salt and pepper to taste

• Lemon wedges for garnish (optional)

Instructions:

- Preheat the oven to 400°F (200°C) and line a baking sheet with parchment paper.

- Place the salmon fillet in the center of the baking sheet and surround it with chopped mixed vegetables.

- Drizzle olive oil over the salmon and vegetables, then sprinkle with dried Italian seasoning, salt, and pepper.

- Bake in the preheated oven for 15-20 minutes, or until the salmon is cooked through and flakes easily with a fork, and the vegetables are tender.

- Remove from the oven and let it rest for a few minutes.

- Serve the baked salmon and roasted vegetables hot, with lemon wedges on the side for garnish if desired.

Health Benefits:

- Salmon is rich in omega-3 fatty acids, which may help reduce inflammation and support heart health.

- Mixed vegetables provide vitamins, minerals, and antioxidants while being low in potassium, supporting overall health and immune function.

- Olive oil is a source of heart-healthy monounsaturated fats and adds flavor to the dish.

Preparation Time: Approximately 25 minutes.

2. Quinoa Stuffed Bell Peppers:

Ingredients:

- 2 large bell peppers, halved and seeds removed
- 1/2 cup quinoa, rinsed
- 1 cup low-sodium vegetable broth
- 1/2 cup cooked black beans, rinsed and drained
- 1/2 cup diced tomatoes
- 1/4 cup diced red onion
- 1/4 cup diced zucchini
- 1/4 teaspoon garlic powder
- 1/4 teaspoon ground cumin
- Salt and pepper to taste
- Fresh cilantro for garnish (optional)

Instructions:

- Preheat the oven to 375°F (190°C) and lightly grease a baking dish.

- In a saucepan, bring the vegetable broth to a boil, then add the rinsed quinoa.

- Reduce the heat to low, cover, and simmer for 15-20 minutes, or until the quinoa is cooked and the liquid is absorbed.

- In a large mixing bowl, combine cooked quinoa, black beans, diced tomatoes, diced red onion, diced zucchini, garlic powder, ground cumin, salt, and pepper.

- Fill each bell pepper half with the quinoa mixture, pressing down gently to pack it in.

- Place the stuffed bell peppers in the prepared baking dish.

- Cover the dish with aluminum foil and bake in the preheated oven for 25-30 minutes, or until the bell peppers are tender.

- Remove from the oven and let it cool slightly before serving.

- Garnish with fresh cilantro if desired.

Health Benefits:

- Quinoa is a gluten-free whole grain rich in protein and fiber, promoting satiety and digestive health.

- Black beans provide plant-based protein and fiber, supporting muscle health and stabilizing blood sugar levels.

- Bell peppers are low in potassium and provide vitamin C, antioxidants, and fiber, promoting overall health and immune function.

Preparation Time: Approximately 45 minutes.

3. Baked Chicken and Vegetable Casserole:

Ingredients:

- 2 boneless, skinless chicken breasts

- 2 cups diced potatoes

- 1 cup chopped carrots

- 1 cup chopped broccoli florets

- 1/4 cup low-sodium chicken broth

- 2 tablespoons olive oil

- 1 teaspoon garlic powder

- 1 teaspoon dried thyme

- Salt and pepper to taste

- Fresh parsley for garnish (optional)

Instructions:

- Preheat the oven to 375°F (190°C) and lightly grease a baking dish.

- Place the diced potatoes, chopped carrots, and broccoli florets in the baking dish.

- Drizzle olive oil and low-sodium chicken broth over the vegetables, then sprinkle with garlic powder, dried thyme, salt, and pepper. Toss to coat evenly.

- Place the boneless, skinless chicken breasts on top of the vegetables.

- Season the chicken breasts with salt, pepper, and additional garlic powder if desired.

- Cover the baking dish with aluminum foil and bake in the preheated oven for 30-35 minutes, or until the chicken is cooked through and the vegetables are tender.

- Remove from the oven and let it rest for a few minutes before serving.

- Garnish with fresh parsley if desired.

Health Benefits:

- Chicken breasts are a lean source of protein and provide essential amino acids for muscle maintenance and repair.

- Potatoes, carrots, and broccoli provide vitamins, minerals, and antioxidants while being low in potassium, supporting overall health and immune function.

- Olive oil adds heart-healthy monounsaturated fats and enhances the flavor of the dish.

Preparation Time: Approximately 45 minutes.

4. Turkey and Quinoa Stuffed Acorn Squash:

Ingredients:

- 2 acorn squash, halved and seeds removed

- 1/2 cup quinoa, rinsed

- 1 cup low-sodium vegetable broth

- 1/2 pound lean ground turkey

- 1/4 cup diced onion

- 1/4 cup diced celery

- 1/4 cup diced bell pepper

- 1 clove garlic, minced

- 1 teaspoon dried sage

- Salt and pepper to taste

- Olive oil for drizzling

Instructions:

• Preheat the oven to 400°F (200°C) and line a baking sheet with parchment paper.

• Place the acorn squash halves, cut side down, on the prepared baking sheet. Bake for 25-30 minutes, or until the squash is tender.

• In a saucepan, bring the vegetable broth to a boil, then add the rinsed quinoa. Reduce the heat to low, cover, and simmer for 15-20 minutes, or until the quinoa is cooked and the liquid is absorbed.

• In a skillet, heat olive oil over medium heat. Add diced onion, celery, bell pepper, and minced garlic, and cook until softened.

• Add lean ground turkey to the skillet and cook until browned and cooked through.

• Stir in cooked quinoa and dried sage, and season with salt and pepper to taste.

• Fill each baked acorn squash half with the turkey and quinoa mixture.

• Drizzle with a little olive oil and return to the oven. Bake for an additional 10-15 minutes, or until heated through.

• Serve hot and enjoy!

Health Benefits:

• Acorn squash is low in potassium and provides vitamins A and C, antioxidants, and fiber, promoting overall health and immune function.

• Quinoa is a gluten-free whole grain rich in protein and fiber, promoting satiety and digestive health.

• Lean ground turkey is a good source of protein and provides essential amino acids for muscle maintenance and repair.

Preparation Time: Approximately 60 minutes.

5. Lemon Herb Baked Cod:

Ingredients:

• 2 cod fillets (4-6 ounces each)

• 1 lemon, thinly sliced

• 2 tablespoons chopped fresh parsley

• 2 tablespoons olive oil

• 1 clove garlic, minced

• 1 teaspoon dried oregano

• Salt and pepper to taste

Instructions:

- Preheat the oven to 400°F (200°C) and line a baking dish with parchment paper.

- Place the cod fillets in the baking dish and season with salt and pepper.

- In a small bowl, whisk together olive oil, minced garlic, and dried oregano.

- Drizzle the olive oil mixture over the cod fillets.

- Arrange lemon slices on top of the cod fillets and sprinkle with chopped fresh parsley.

- Bake in the preheated oven for 12-15 minutes, or until the cod is cooked through and flakes easily with a fork.

- Serve hot with your choice of side dishes.

Health Benefits:

- Cod is a lean source of protein and provides omega-3 fatty acids, which may help reduce inflammation and support heart health.

- Lemons add flavor and provide vitamin C, antioxidants, and citric acid, which may help prevent kidney stones.

- Olive oil is rich in heart-healthy monounsaturated fats and enhances the flavor of the dish.

Preparation Time: Approximately 20 minutes.

6. Vegetable and Lentil Curry:

Ingredients:

- 1 cup dried green lentils, rinsed and drained

- 2 cups low-sodium vegetable broth

- 1 tablespoon olive oil

- 1 onion, diced

- 2 cloves garlic, minced

- 1 tablespoon curry powder

- 1 teaspoon ground cumin

- 1 teaspoon ground turmeric

- 1 can (14 ounces) diced tomatoes, undrained

- 2 cups chopped mixed vegetables (such as bell peppers, carrots, and spinach)

- Salt and pepper to taste

- Fresh cilantro for garnish (optional)

Instructions:

- In a saucepan, combine dried green lentils and low-sodium vegetable broth. Bring to a boil, then reduce heat, cover, and simmer for 20-25 minutes, or until the lentils are tender.

- In a large skillet, heat olive oil over medium heat. Add diced onion and minced garlic, and cook until softened.

- Stir in curry powder, ground cumin, and ground turmeric, and cook for 1-2 minutes, until fragrant.

- Add diced tomatoes (with their juices) and chopped mixed vegetables to the skillet, and stir to combine.

- Cook for 5-7 minutes, or until the vegetables are tender.

- Stir in cooked lentils and simmer for an additional 5 minutes to allow the flavors to meld.

- Season with salt and pepper to taste.

- Serve hot, garnished with fresh cilantro if desired, and enjoy!

Health Benefits:

- Lentils are a good source of plant-based protein and fiber, promoting satiety and digestive health.

- Mixed vegetables provide vitamins, minerals, and antioxidants while being low in potassium, supporting overall health and immune function.

- Curry powder, cumin, and turmeric add flavor and provide anti-inflammatory properties.

Preparation Time: Approximately 45 minutes.

7. Quinoa and Vegetable Stir-Fry:

Ingredients:

- 1/2 cup quinoa, rinsed

- 1 cup low-sodium vegetable broth

- 1 tablespoon olive oil

- 1 onion, diced

- 2 cloves garlic, minced

- 1 cup mixed vegetables (such as bell peppers, broccoli, and carrots), chopped

- 1 tablespoon low-sodium soy sauce

- 1 teaspoon sesame oil

- 1 tablespoon chopped green onions (optional)

- Salt and pepper to taste

Instructions:

• In a saucepan, bring the vegetable broth to a boil, then add the rinsed quinoa. Reduce the heat to low, cover, and simmer for 15-20 minutes, or until the quinoa is cooked and the liquid is absorbed.

• In a large skillet or wok, heat olive oil over medium heat. Add diced onion and minced garlic, and cook until softened.

• Add chopped mixed vegetables to the skillet and stir-fry until tender-crisp.

• Stir in cooked quinoa, low-sodium soy sauce, and sesame oil, and toss to combine.

• Cook for an additional 2-3 minutes, until heated through.

• Season with salt and pepper to taste.

• Garnish with chopped green onions if desired.

• Serve hot and enjoy!

Health Benefits:

• Quinoa is a gluten-free whole grain rich in protein and fiber, promoting satiety and digestive health.

• Mixed vegetables offer a variety of vitamins, minerals, and antioxidants while being low in potassium, supporting overall health and immune function.

- Olive oil provides heart-healthy monounsaturated fats, while sesame oil adds flavor and aroma to the dish.

Preparation Time: Approximately 30 minutes.

8. Baked Eggplant Parmesan:

Ingredients:

- 1 large eggplant, sliced into rounds
- 1 cup whole wheat breadcrumbs
- 1/4 cup grated Parmesan cheese
- 1 teaspoon dried oregano
- 1 teaspoon dried basil
- 2 eggs, beaten
- 1 cup marinara sauce (low-sodium or homemade)
- 1 cup shredded mozzarella cheese
- Fresh basil leaves for garnish (optional)
- Salt and pepper to taste

Instructions:

- Preheat the oven to 400°F (200°C) and line a baking sheet with parchment paper.

- In a shallow dish, combine whole wheat breadcrumbs, grated Parmesan cheese, dried oregano, and dried basil. Season with salt and pepper.

- Dip each eggplant slice into the beaten eggs, then dredge in the breadcrumb mixture, coating evenly.

- Place the coated eggplant slices on the prepared baking sheet.

- Bake in the preheated oven for 20-25 minutes, or until the eggplant is golden brown and tender.

- Remove from the oven and spoon marinara sauce over each eggplant slice.

- Sprinkle shredded mozzarella cheese on top of the marinara sauce.

- Return to the oven and bake for an additional 10 minutes, or until the cheese is melted and bubbly.

- Garnish with fresh basil leaves if desired.

- Serve hot and enjoy!

Health Benefits:

- Eggplant is low in potassium and provides fiber, antioxidants, and phytonutrients, supporting digestive health and reducing inflammation.

- Whole wheat breadcrumbs offer complex carbohydrates and fiber, promoting satiety and digestive health.

- Marinara sauce provides lycopene and vitamins from tomatoes while being low in sodium.

Preparation Time: Approximately 45 minutes.

9. Lemon Garlic Shrimp with Asparagus:

Ingredients:

- 8 ounces shrimp, peeled and deveined
- 1 bunch asparagus, trimmed and cut into bite-sized pieces
- 2 tablespoons olive oil
- 3 cloves garlic, minced
- 1 lemon, juiced and zested
- 1 tablespoon chopped fresh parsley
- Salt and pepper to taste

Instructions:

- In a large skillet, heat olive oil over medium heat. Add minced garlic and cook until fragrant, about 1 minute.

- Add shrimp to the skillet and cook until pink and opaque, about 2-3 minutes per side.

- Add asparagus to the skillet and cook until tender-crisp, about 4-5 minutes.

- Stir in lemon juice and zest, and chopped fresh parsley. Season with salt and pepper to taste.

Cook for an additional minute to allow the flavors to meld.

Remove from heat and serve hot.

Health Benefits:

Shrimp is a good source of protein and provides essential nutrients such as selenium and vitamin B12.

Asparagus is low in potassium and provides vitamins A, C, and K, as well as folate and fiber.

Garlic and lemon add flavor without adding extra sodium, making this dish kidney-friendly.

Preparation Time: Approximately 20 minutes.

10. Turkey and Vegetable Skillet:

Ingredients:

- 1 pound ground turkey

- 1 onion, diced

- 2 cloves garlic, minced

- 2 cups diced mixed vegetables (such as bell peppers, zucchini, and carrots)

- 1 can (14 ounces) low-sodium diced tomatoes, drained

- 1 teaspoon dried basil

- 1 teaspoon dried oregano

- Salt and pepper to taste

Instructions:

- In a large skillet, cook ground turkey over medium heat until browned and cooked through, breaking it apart with a spoon.

- Add diced onion and minced garlic to the skillet and cook until softened, about 3-4 minutes.

- Stir in diced mixed vegetables and cook until tender, about 5-6 minutes.

- Add drained diced tomatoes, dried basil, and dried oregano to the skillet. Season with salt and pepper to taste.

- Cook for an additional 2-3 minutes to allow the flavors to meld.

- Remove from heat and serve hot.

Health Benefits:

• Ground turkey is a lean source of protein and provides essential nutrients such as selenium and vitamin B12.

• Mixed vegetables offer a variety of vitamins, minerals, and antioxidants while being low in potassium.

• Dried herbs add flavor without adding extra sodium, making this dish kidney-friendly.

Preparation Time: Approximately 30 minutes.

CKD Stage 3 Snack Recipes

1. Baked Sweet Potato Chips:

Ingredients:

• 2 medium sweet potatoes, washed and peeled

• 1 tablespoon olive oil

• Salt to taste

Instructions:

• Preheat the oven to 375°F (190°C) and line a baking sheet with parchment paper.

• Using a mandoline slicer or sharp knife, slice the sweet potatoes thinly and evenly.

- Place the sweet potato slices in a bowl and toss with olive oil until evenly coated.

- Arrange the sweet potato slices in a single layer on the prepared baking sheet.

- Sprinkle with salt to taste.

- Bake in the preheated oven for 15-20 minutes, flipping halfway through, until the chips are golden brown and crispy.

- Remove from the oven and let cool before serving.

- Enjoy as a crispy and nutritious snack!

Health Benefits:

Sweet potatoes are rich in vitamins A and C, potassium, and fiber, providing essential nutrients while being low in phosphorus and sodium.

Olive oil adds heart-healthy monounsaturated fats and enhances the flavor of the chips.

Preparation Time: Approximately 30 minutes.

2. Greek Yogurt with Berries and Almonds:
Ingredients:

- 1/2 cup plain Greek yogurt

- 1/4 cup mixed berries (such as blueberries, strawberries, and raspberries)

- 1 tablespoon chopped almonds

Instructions:

- In a small bowl, spoon Greek yogurt.

- Top with mixed berries and chopped almonds.

- Serve immediately and enjoy as a refreshing and protein-rich snack!

Health Benefits:

Greek yogurt is high in protein and calcium, supporting muscle health and bone strength.

- Berries are rich in antioxidants and fiber, promoting heart health and digestion.

- Almonds provide healthy fats, vitamin E, and magnesium, supporting overall health and well-being.

Preparation Time: Approximately 5 minutes.

3. Cucumber and Hummus Bites:

Ingredients:

- 1 large cucumber

- 1/4 cup hummus

- Fresh parsley or dill for garnish (optional)

Instructions:

- Wash the cucumber and slice it into thick rounds.

- Use a small spoon or melon baller to scoop out a shallow well in each cucumber slice.

- Fill each cucumber well with a small dollop of hummus.

- Garnish with fresh parsley or dill if desired.

- Arrange the cucumber and hummus bites on a serving platter.

- Serve immediately and enjoy as a refreshing and protein-rich snack!

Health Benefits:

- Cucumbers are low in potassium and provide hydration and a refreshing crunch.

- Hummus is made from chickpeas, which are a good source of plant-based protein and fiber, supporting digestive health and satiety.

Preparation Time: Approximately 10 minutes.

4. Apple and Almond Butter Slices:

Ingredients:

- 1 apple, cored and thinly sliced

- 2 tablespoons almond butter
- 1 tablespoon chopped almonds
- Cinnamon for sprinkling (optional)

Instructions:

- Core the apple and slice it into thin rounds.
- Spread almond butter on each apple slice.
- Sprinkle chopped almonds on top of the almond butter.
- Optional: Sprinkle with cinnamon for added flavor.
- Arrange the apple and almond butter slices on a serving plate.
- Serve immediately and enjoy as a nutritious and satisfying snack!

Health Benefits:

- Apples are low in potassium and provide fiber, antioxidants, and vitamins, promoting heart health and digestion.
- Almond butter is a good source of healthy fats, protein, and vitamin E, supporting overall health and well-being.

Preparation Time: Approximately 5 minutes.

5. Rice Cake with Avocado and Tomato:

Ingredients:

- 1 rice cake

- 1/4 ripe avocado, mashed

- 1 small tomato, sliced

- Pinch of sea salt

- Optional: Sprinkle of black pepper or red pepper flakes

Instructions:

- Spread mashed avocado evenly on top of the rice cake.

- Place tomato slices on top of the avocado layer.

- Sprinkle with a pinch of sea salt.

- Optional: Add a sprinkle of black pepper or red pepper flakes for added flavor.

- Serve immediately and enjoy as a light and nutritious snack!

Health Benefits:

- Rice cakes are low in sodium and provide a crunchy base for the snack.

- Avocado is rich in heart-healthy monounsaturated fats, vitamins, and minerals, supporting overall health and satiety.

- Tomatoes are low in potassium and provide vitamins A and C, antioxidants, and lycopene, promoting heart health and reducing inflammation.

Preparation Time: Approximately 5 minutes.

6. Cottage Cheese and Pineapple Spears:

Ingredients:

- 1/2 cup low-fat cottage cheese

- 1/2 cup fresh pineapple chunks

- Wooden skewers or toothpicks

Instructions:

- Thread pineapple chunks onto wooden skewers or toothpicks.

- Serve alongside a small bowl of low-fat cottage cheese.

- Enjoy alternating bites of pineapple and cottage cheese for a refreshing and protein-rich snack!

Health Benefits:

- Cottage cheese is high in protein and calcium, supporting muscle health and bone strength.

• Pineapple is low in potassium and provides vitamin C, manganese, and bromelain, promoting digestion and immune function.

Preparation Time: Approximately 5 minutes.

7. Tuna Cucumber Bites:

Ingredients:

- 1 cucumber

- 1 can (5 ounces) tuna, drained

- 2 tablespoons Greek yogurt

- 1 tablespoon chopped fresh dill

- 1 teaspoon lemon juice

- Salt and pepper to taste

Instructions:

- Wash the cucumber and slice it into thick rounds.

- In a small bowl, mix together drained tuna, Greek yogurt, chopped fresh dill, lemon juice, salt, and pepper.

- Place a small spoonful of the tuna mixture on top of each cucumber slice.

- Serve immediately and enjoy as a protein-rich and refreshing snack!

Health Benefits:

• Cucumbers are low in potassium and provide hydration and a refreshing crunch.

• Tuna is a lean source of protein and provides essential nutrients such as omega-3 fatty acids, supporting heart health and muscle function.

• Greek yogurt adds protein and calcium while being low in phosphorus, supporting bone health and digestion.

Preparation Time: Approximately 10 minutes.

8. Rice Paper Spring Rolls:

Ingredients:

• 4 rice paper wrappers

• 1 cup shredded lettuce

• 1/2 cup thinly sliced cucumber

• 1/2 cup matchstick carrots

• 1/2 cup cooked shrimp, chopped

• Fresh mint leaves

• Dipping sauce (low-sodium soy sauce or sweet chili sauce), for serving

Instructions:

• Fill a shallow dish with warm water.

• Dip one rice paper wrapper into the warm water for a few seconds until softened.

• Place the softened rice paper wrapper on a clean work surface.

• Layer shredded lettuce, sliced cucumber, matchstick carrots, chopped cooked shrimp, and fresh mint leaves on the bottom third of the rice paper wrapper.

• Fold the bottom of the wrapper over the filling, then fold in the sides, and roll tightly to enclose the filling.

• Repeat with the remaining rice paper wrappers and filling ingredients.

• Serve the spring rolls with dipping sauce on the side.

• Enjoy these light and flavorful spring rolls as a nutritious snack!

Health Benefits:

• Rice paper wrappers are low in potassium and provide a gluten-free and low-calorie wrapper for the spring rolls.

• Vegetables such as lettuce, cucumber, and carrots provide fiber, vitamins, and minerals, promoting digestion and overall health.

- Shrimp adds protein and essential nutrients such as selenium and vitamin B12, supporting muscle health and immune function.

Preparation Time: Approximately 20 minutes.

9. Egg Salad Lettuce Wraps:

Ingredients:

- 2 hard-boiled eggs, chopped
- 2 tablespoons Greek yogurt
- 1 teaspoon Dijon mustard
- 1 tablespoon chopped chives
- Salt and pepper to taste
- 4 large lettuce leaves (such as romaine or butterhead)

Instructions:

- In a bowl, combine chopped hard-boiled eggs, Greek yogurt, Dijon mustard, chopped chives, salt, and pepper.
- Mix well until all ingredients are evenly combined.
- Place a spoonful of the egg salad mixture onto each lettuce leaf.
- Roll up the lettuce leaves to form wraps.

• Serve immediately and enjoy these protein-rich and low-carb snacks!

Health Benefits:

• Hard-boiled eggs are a good source of protein and provide essential nutrients such as vitamin D and choline, supporting bone health and brain function.

• Greek yogurt adds protein and calcium while being low in phosphorus and sodium, promoting digestive health and bone strength.

• Lettuce leaves provide hydration and fiber, supporting digestion and overall health.

Preparation Time: Approximately 15 minutes.

10. Caprese Skewers:

Ingredients:

• 12 cherry tomatoes

• 12 fresh mozzarella balls

• 12 fresh basil leaves

• Balsamic glaze for drizzling (optional)

• Wooden skewers

Instructions:

- Thread one cherry tomato, one fresh mozzarella ball, and one fresh basil leaf onto each wooden skewer.

- Repeat until all ingredients are used.

- Arrange the skewers on a serving platter.

- Optional: Drizzle with balsamic glaze for added flavor.

- Serve immediately and enjoy these flavorful and protein-rich snacks!

Health Benefits:

- Cherry tomatoes are low in potassium and provide vitamins A and C, antioxidants, and lycopene, promoting heart health and reducing inflammation.

- Fresh mozzarella is lower in sodium compared to aged cheeses and provides protcin and calcium, supporting muscle health and bone strength.

- Fresh basil adds flavor and aroma while providing antioxidants and anti-inflammatory properties.

Preparation Time: Approximately 10 minutes.

CONCLUSION

Common Concerns About Diet and CKD Stage 3

Individuals with Chronic Kidney Disease (CKD) Stage 3 often have various concerns related to their diet, as nutrition plays a crucial role in managing the condition and slowing disease progression. Here are common concerns about diet and CKD Stage 3:

1. Protein Intake:

One common concern is how to manage protein intake. Individuals with CKD Stage 3 are typically advised to limit their protein intake to reduce the burden on the kidneys and minimize the accumulation of waste products in the body. However, ensuring an adequate intake of high-quality protein is essential for maintaining muscle mass and overall health.

2. Sodium (Salt) Restriction:

Another concern is managing sodium intake. Excess sodium can lead to fluid retention and hypertension, which are common complications of CKD. Individuals with CKD Stage 3 are often advised to limit their sodium intake to control blood pressure and reduce the risk of fluid overload and swelling (edema).

3. Potassium and Phosphorus Levels: Managing potassium and phosphorus levels in the diet is also a concern for individuals with

CKD Stage 3. High levels of potassium and phosphorus in the blood can lead to complications such as abnormal heart rhythms and bone disorders. Monitoring and limiting the intake of potassium- and phosphorus-rich foods, such as bananas, oranges, dairy products, and processed meats, is essential.

4. Fluid Intake:

Fluid management is another common concern. Individuals with CKD Stage 3 may experience fluid retention, which can lead to swelling, high blood pressure, and shortness of breath. Monitoring fluid intake and adhering to fluid restrictions recommended by healthcare providers is crucial for preventing fluid overload and alleviating symptoms.

5. Micronutrient Deficiencies:

Concerns about micronutrient deficiencies are also prevalent. CKD can affect the body's ability to absorb and utilize certain vitamins and minerals, such as vitamin D, calcium, iron, and B vitamins. Ensuring adequate intake of these nutrients through diet and supplementation is important for preventing deficiencies and supporting overall health.

Addressing these common concerns about diet and CKD Stage 3 requires careful monitoring, individualized nutrition counseling, and adherence to dietary recommendations provided by healthcare providers and registered dietitians specializing in renal nutrition. With proper guidance and education, individuals with CKD Stage 3 can effectively manage their diet to support kidney health and improve overall well-being.

Lifestyle Adjustments for Better Kidney Health

Making lifestyle adjustments is essential for promoting better kidney health, especially for individuals with Chronic Kidney Disease (CKD) or those at risk of developing kidney problems. Here are key lifestyle adjustments for better kidney health:

1. Maintain a Healthy Weight:

Excess weight can increase the risk of developing conditions such as diabetes and hypertension, which are leading causes of CKD.

Adopting a balanced diet and engaging in regular physical activity can help achieve and maintain a healthy weight, reducing the risk of kidney disease progression.

2. Follow a Balanced Diet:

A balanced diet that is low in sodium, saturated fats, and processed foods and rich in fruits, vegetables, whole grains, and lean proteins is beneficial for kidney health.

Following dietary recommendations tailored to individual needs, such as limiting phosphorus and potassium intake for individuals with CKD, can help manage symptoms and slow disease progression.

3. Stay Hydrated:

Drinking an adequate amount of fluids, primarily water, is important for maintaining kidney function and preventing dehydration. However, individuals with CKD may need to monitor their fluid intake closely, as excessive fluid intake can lead to fluid retention and worsen kidney function.

4. Monitor Blood Pressure:

High blood pressure is a leading cause of kidney damage. Monitoring blood pressure regularly and taking steps to keep it within a healthy range, such as following a low-sodium diet, exercising regularly, and taking prescribed medications, can help protect kidney health.

5. Avoid Smoking and Limit Alcohol Intake:

Smoking and excessive alcohol consumption can impair kidney function and increase the risk of kidney disease. Quitting smoking and limiting alcohol intake can help reduce the risk of kidney damage and improve overall health.

6. Manage Stress:

Chronic stress can contribute to the development and progression of kidney disease. Engaging in stress-reducing activities such as meditation, yoga, deep breathing exercises, and hobbies can help promote better kidney health and overall well-being.

7. Get Regular Exercise:

Regular physical activity can help improve cardiovascular health, control weight, and reduce the risk of developing conditions such as diabetes and hypertension, which are risk factors for CKD. Aim for at least 150 minutes of moderate-intensity exercise per week, as recommended by guidelines.

www.ingramcontent.com/pod-product-compliance
Lightning Source LLC
Chambersburg PA
CBHW071949210526
45479CB00003B/870